Schizophrenia
Understanding Symptoms Diagnosis & Treatment

How to deal with a loved one with Schizophrenia

Anthony Wilkenson

Legal Disclaimer

Table of Contents

Important Insight

Schizophrenia has become a recognized psychotic disorder in modern day psychology and research has shown that 1 in 100 people suffer from this disease in some proportion or degree.

It is a dreaded disease and comes as a near death blow to those who are diagnosed with this condition. This fear does not necessarily arise from the scary disease it actually is, but various misconceptions, myths and misunderstanding that surround it.

This disorder has been very thoroughly misunderstood and misrepresented. As a result, there is great confusion and stigma attached to it. This stigma, social pressure, and public opinion have made it very difficult to get the disorder diagnosed, treated or managed.

Persons suffering from schizophrenia or under a risk of being affected by it are very insecure due to this public opinion. There has been so much talk about this psychotic disorder with little or no knowledge about it, that it has spread a rumor about the hopelessness and incurability of it.

This book aims at spreading awareness and information about Schizophrenia and act as a guide for those who want to have a better understanding of this horrible condition.

1: What is Schizophrenia?

Schizophrenia is a mental disorder which alters the way a person perceives this world or its aspects. Schizophrenia makes it difficult for the person who is infected to know the difference between the real and the unreal, or have a clear understanding of reality. They have a hard time establishing a relationship with various things of the world.

It affects the perception to such an extent that a person suffering from it does not know the difference between what is imaginary and what is truly existent.

It leads to false beliefs, hallucinations, auditory misconceptions, anger, frustration, confusion, disturbed thoughts, inaction, extreme emotional disturbances, decreasing/increasing social interaction, biased sense perception etc.

Their loss of contact with the actual world could be severely disturbed, or they may also feel a sense of loss about something which is not understood or known by others, or be suspicious of somebody's activities, or live in constant fear that they are being watched, are under scrutiny, or being harmed.

They may also come up with an object or person they really love or hate and have a totally different opinion about it. Their perception may have no connection at all with reality. And at times, reality holds no relevance to them. They form a world of their own.

They may also develop or acquire weird dressing style or unhygienic habits, be sloppy in their lifestyle or eating habits, have a new way of talking which results from disconnected chain of thoughts.

Paranoia is a common symptom which is characterized by systematized delusions and the projection of personal conflicts. They also have a responsive disorder to conversation with other people.

Memory, retention, expression, articulation, speed of thought processing, day to day activities are affected and there have been patterns of decreasing social interaction and more isolation.

People suffering from schizophrenia are seen with different moods and no two schizophrenic persons are alike. Same disease may affect two individuals with different backgrounds differently and make every individual unique.

Schizophrenia affects normally the younger generation and even children. The symptoms in children are slightly different. However, there is no rule and it may appear to show signs in anybody at any age. Schizophrenic symptoms may be seen in grownups or middle aged people as well even if there were no signs earlier.

Studies have shown that the younger the patient, more severe are the effects of the disease and the condition gets worse with age.

It is also known that men are more chronic and deeply schizophrenic than women, i.e. men make some of the worst cases of schizophrenia ever. These symptoms may be coupled with other disorders like mood swings, depression, anxiety and some other disease.

History of schizophrenia is obscure. Literally the word finds its origin from the Greek words schizein means "to split" and phren means "mind".
It was believed that schizophrenia means to have a split personality and a person hearing voices has another personality who talks to him.

We do not find historical records which could provide evidences of this disease till we heard of the case report of James Tilly Mathews and accounts by Phillipe Pinel which was published in 1809.

This report has been considered as the earliest dependable reference of mental disorders and psychiatric analysis.

Till about the 20th century, there was no clear cut demarcation and definition of schizophrenia and dissociative personalities. Then the famous psychiatrist Kurt Schneider came up with a detailed analysis and symptoms of schizophrenia which distinguished it from split personality disorder and other mental diseases.

This definition and categorization is known as "first rank symptoms" or "Schneider's first rank symptoms". This includes delusions, feeling of being controlled by an external force, thoughts being planted or removed from one's mind, thoughts not remaining private, hearing voices, communicating with these voices, etc.

With the help of latest research, it has been established that schizophrenia does not involve switching personalities or changing himself/herself into somebody else.

It is just a matter of imagination that one's own chatter of the mind sounds or looks like some other person who has been talking to them.

2: Behavioral Tendencies Leading To Schizophrenia

You must have seen cases where Schizophrenia appeared out of nowhere. This is not always so. Sometimes the symptoms exist but too subtle to be noticed, or people may not show any signs publicly.

In such cases when the disease is existent but hidden, then for friends and family it is a sudden case of emergence. Such cases are very dangerous for the person suffering from Schizophrenia, and by the time it comes to our attention, it has already become chronic or it is too late.

Sometimes, people around an individual are too careless to pay attention in the beginning. Even very caring and sensible companions cannot figure out what is wrong.

There have been stories where the friends and family have complained that they knew that their friend/son/daughter/husband/wife was changing but couldn't exactly point out as to what was wrong. The changes are too subtle and slow to be pointed out and given a name.

People ignore it as stress, anger, frustration, or fear and it goes unnoticed for a long period of time till it becomes too stark and pronounced.

People who are at the beginning stage of Schizophrenia often appear slightly eccentric, reclusive, irate, and emotionally upset. Such upsets may be prolonged or short. They may start ignoring their appearance, be untidy, ignore work or responsibilities, start with new way of talking, say weird things, and are indifferent to life and its surroundings.

In some cases they abandon their own hobbies and even start a new one. Performance at work or school deteriorates.

Some very commonly seen behavioral changes indicating one has schizophrenia are:

• Withdrawl from society, suspicion, hostile temperament, withdrawn gaze, and lack of expressions.

• Lack of personal hygiene and cleanliness, untimely and unnecessary expressions of joy or pain - not expressing joy or pain in a normal way.

• Lack of concentration, depression, forgetfulness and sleep disorders: Insomnia or over sleeping.

• Changed way of speaking or using a different vocabulary, peculiar statements, extreme reactions to praise, blame and criticism.

Some facts about schizophrenia

• Schizophrenia is often confused with "split personality" or "multiple personality disorder". Schizophrenia is more common than multiple or split personalities. Schizophrenic individuals are just one person and one personality.

• It is not a rare disorder, it is a common disorder and 1 in 100 persons stand a chance of being schizophrenic.

• Schizophrenic persons are not dangerous as is the case with some other mental disorders. They may commit an act of violence in a sudden spurt of anger; otherwise they are mostly delusive and depressed. They do not hurt or become a threat to others.

• It is not incurable. Chronic patients may take a long time to respond to treatment, but it's not an incurable disease. It is a time taking process to treat them but they are also capable of leading a normal life, perform normal functions and be an active part of family and community.

Two categories of symptoms have been described; positive and negative.

Positive symptoms

Positive symptoms are those which are not felt or experienced all the time. It may occur from time to time like delusions, speech and thought disorders, irrational behavior, or visual or auditory hallucinations which are also known as "manifestations of psychosis".

These people stand a better chance of getting cured and respond very well to treatment.

Negative symptoms

Negative symptoms are somewhat different. They include lack of poor emotional responses, inability to feel joy or pain, lack of desire to interact with others, work, study, lack of motivation, depression, and functional disability.

Such patients have poor adjustment capabilities before the onset of the disease. Their response to treatment is very poor and slow and chances of recovery are also meager.

There are 5 major categories of symptoms

Delusions are found in 90% cases of schizophrenia. Delusion is a belief which is held against all odds, evidence and analysis. Delusions in schizophrenic patients are bizarre, weird, illogical and fanciful.

- Delusions of persecution are cases where the patients believes that some person or group of persons are "out to get him/her." These persons or group of persons are sometimes totally imaginative.

There once was a case when a patient felt that the persecutors of Jesus are out to poison him with Mercury and refused to eat anything which was not cooked directly by him.

He refused to eat packed or frozen foods, didn't eat vegetables from the market, and never ate at hotels.

- Delusions of control makes a patient think that he/she is being controlled by an outside or supernatural force. There was a case where the patient felt that some force has hypnotized and gained control of his mind and his thoughts are no longer private.

He even felt that they are planting thoughts in his mind and using him as medium to get things done. They are stealing his thoughts and claiming it as their creation.

- Delusions of reference happen when a person suffering from schizophrenia believes that a movie or a news telecast is indicating towards a message specifically meant for him. A patient used to watch nightly news telecast everyday and picks up key words to decide upon the menu for dinner. He believed that GOD was talking to him through that telecast.

- Delusions of grandeur is seen where people believe that they are somebody else, somebody great like Jesus Christ or Alexander the Great, or believe that they are blessed with some special power which no one else has.

They believe that they can change the sequence of events or even fly. Once a man hurt himself while trying to fly off from his 5th floor house balcony and when he failed he claimed that a demon has snatched away his power.

There have been cases where the person felt that he was the king of an area and asked everybody to obey him.

Hallucinations

Hallucination is a state where a voice, vision or sensations felt by a person out of his/her imagination is believed to be real, but in reality, they only exist in his head.

Hallucination may have all the five senses involved or it could be just one or two senses in action. They hear voices talking to them, sitting in front of them, or walking or sleeping with them. In a severe case they may even feel it.

Most of the time, these voices are of people they know and at times of strangers. Auditory hallucinations occur because people misinterpret the voice and chatter off their own mind as others' talks. They even send and receive messages through them. They are meaningful to the person who hears it and it worsens when a person is alone.

There was once a person suffering from schizophrenia that laid a table for two at every meal time and always served coffee in two cups. Had her share first, then swapped places and had the other person's share and went on to believe that she lived and ate with her husband who had been dead for years.

People saw her eating twice from two different plates but nobody could convince her of the reality.

Disorganized and non-sensible speech

- A schizophrenic has fragmented thoughts and is evident in his/her way of talking also. They cannot maintain a proper synchronized chain of thoughts and as a result, the speech is also fragmented and disconnected.

They start with a topic and end with something entirely different, give unrelated answers to questions, speak nonsense things.

- They change topics quickly, shifting from one to another without a gap.

- They have a vocabulary of their own and it makes sense only to them. It may also have some similar sounding words which make no sense as a statement.

- They are very repetitive and may go on telling the same thing over and over again and are not aware of the repetition or incoherence.

Irrational behavior

- The action and behavior is not goal oriented. They do a task for some reason which is only understood by them and not others. They cannot take care of themselves.

- Normal functions become disturbed and they cannot do it properly.

- Emotional responses are unpredictable and peculiar.

- Behavior is bizarre and weird and there is no control on impulses.

Negative symptoms

These negative symptoms are the most difficult cases to be treated.

- There may be blank faces where there are no expressions, flat voice and no eye contact.

- No motivation and zeal, and there is no enthusiasm about anything.

- Speaking in a mono tone, unaware of the social environment, disconnected replies and inability to communicate.

These are some of the most commonly found symptoms and signs of schizophrenia. It is not necessary that all symptoms will be positively present in a patient. Some may be seen, others not, that too in varying degrees.

Symptoms are also indicative of how serious the case of schizophrenia, which play a vital role in marking diagnosis, treatment and improvement. Watch out for any such signs but do not be afraid if you find some. It may not be schizophrenia but some other psychotic disorder.

3: Early Diagnosis of Schizophrenia can really Help

In order to successfully diagnose Schizophrenia, some modern criteria has been recognized. There is no objective test to ensure a 100% diagnosis. These criteria use the self-assessed feelings and experiences of the persons or some abnormality that they feel that has been bothering them at behavioral level.

Once analyzed, a clinical analysis is conducted by experts and professionals. The symptoms have to reach a serious level before they can get detected.

DSM-5

DSM-5 is the new criteria for diagnosing schizophrenia. According to this criteria, a person has to show under clinical supervision for a period of one month, symptoms which have been largely associated with schizophrenia, like hallucinations, delusions, hearing voices, change in behavior which has a significant impact on social and professional spaces, or the negative symptoms like social withdrawal, disinterest or severely disorganized thoughts or speech, and these symptoms must be in existence in six months of recent history.

If an individual is seen as undergoing any of these behavioral disorders, then he/she is considered to be suffering from some form of schizophrenia.

- Some terms and types like "paranoid schizophrenia" and "catatonia" are no longer considered relevant as subtypes of schizophrenia.

- Schneider's first-rank symptoms are not considered relevant any longer.

- Schizoaffective disorder is demarcated from schizophrenia to avoid confusion between the two.

- There is an eight point assessment report like ensuring whether delusions, hallucinations and mania is a part of the individual's behavior to diagnose the disease accurately.

European countries use ICD-10 criteria to ascertain Schizophrenia. The DSM analysis is used in the United States and many such criteria are in prevalence around the world with slight variations.

If disorders have been persisting for more than a month and less than six months, then the patient is treated for Schizophreniform disorders.

Psychological disturbances lasting for less than a month are categorized as brief psychotic disorders. This person is treated for schizoaffective disorder. Schizophrenia is not considered present if there is an occurrence of pervasive developmental disorder without hallucinations and delusions.

DSM-5 has defined five subtypes of schizophrenia which is accepted in the USA.

1. Paranoid type patients feel hallucinations and delusions but do not have thought disorder or disorganized behavior. They may be delusive in a persecutory or grandiose way, jealousy or even religiosity has been seen.

2. Disorganized type has flat affect and thought disorders are seen.

3. Undifferentiated type subjects have psychotic symptoms but other symptoms like paranoia, disorganized thoughts or catatonic disorders are not found.

4. Residual type has positive symptoms in low intensity and they are not very severe.

5. Catatonic type subjects may be immobile or highly active and agitated without a purpose or cause.

The ICD-10 has defined two more categories:

1. Post Schizophrenic Depression is a kind of depression which a patient recently recovered from schizophrenia faces; it is an aftermath effect of the disease and has some minor symptoms of schizophrenia still in existence.

2. Simple Schizophrenia is a kind when there has been no history of psychotic disorders but there is a developmental tendency in negative symptoms.

Psychotic symptoms are present in other mental disorders like the bipolar disorder, borderline personality disorder, anxiety disorder and avoidant personality disorder and that is why it becomes absolutely imperative to diagnose and look for other symptoms of schizophrenia before starting the treatment.

There has been a general pattern of Obsessive Compulsive Disorder (OCD) being found in schizophrenic patients which is more than a mere coincidence.

There are ways to arrive at a conclusion and ascertain that a person is suffering from schizophrenia. Psychiatric evaluation is done by asking a series of questions to the patient and his loved ones.

Having the knowledge about the mental history of the patient and their family is a big plus. A patient is also checked for physical diseases, in case one of the physical diseases is causing a mental disorder.

There are no laboratory tests for schizophrenia. However, physical tests help in ascertaining the physical health of the body which at times causes a mental illness. Some brain scans may help as there are some abnormalities which result in schizophrenia or some other disease.

When it is ensured that no other physical problem, drug abuse or illness is causing the hallucinations, delusions and other disorders, it is finally decided that the subject is a patient of schizophrenia.

Effects of Schizophrenia

- Such patients withdraw themselves and their disturbed relationships with family and friends.

- Their daily life is severely affected and day-to-day functioning becomes irregular and peculiar.

- The condition of such a subject is so disturbed and their will power is so weak, they easily turn to drugs or alcohol, and the temptations are too great to resist. A restless state of mind also makes them seek solace in intoxicants.

- Chances of suicide increases. There are patients who talk of suicide and as a result, near and dear ones become alert. However, there are some who are very quiet about their thoughts. In such cases, it is very difficult to figure out what is going on in their head. The end result is they commit suicide without warning.

4: Factors Responsible For Causing Schizophrenia

There have been many theories that have been proposed by psychologists and experts as probable causes of schizophrenia. Some of them have been found to be very potent and highly probable.

Others just look like a remote possibility, and there are some minor ones which have not been found as direct causes, but scientists feel that there is some connection. A valid relationship is yet to be established, but a relationship is definitely felt and seen.

Genetic factors

Genes have been known to playing an active role in schizophrenia. It is difficult to ascertain the exact effect because there are heavy variations.

People who have a first-degree relative suffering from schizophrenia have 6.5% more chances acquiring it than others. Monozygotic twins have 40% or more chance. If one of the parents are affected, the risk is 13% or more.

The figures surely look scary to people who have a history of schizophrenia and given the above facts, a direct relationship between schizophrenia and genes cannot be ignored.

There are some common genetic traits which are found in bipolar disorder and schizophrenia. It leads to some overlaps which makes it difficult to point the ones indicating towards schizophrenia

But there is a heavy variation in the genetic traits, as some genetic indicators are very common in mental disorders. Such heavy and multiple variations make it difficult to detect the genetic aspect of this disease.

- There have been evidence of genetic traits being responsible for language development and development of human nature, but these ideas are in its infancy stage and nothing worthwhile has been established until now.

Environmental causes

Environmental factors have been found playing a very vital role in the development of these diseases. The living environment or even prenatal stressors have been found as contributory factors.

If the mother has been constantly in stress or threat while expecting, such children have a greater risk of attracting mental disorders or being psychotic. Parenting has no direct connection with the disease.

However, children with supportive parents are less likely to have disorders. Children with abusive or hostile parents are at a greater risk due to the emotional trauma and lack of emotional support suffered by them.

There are children who suffer some kind of childhood trauma, separation from parents at a young age or they are bullied and mistreated. Such children have a chance of developing psychotic tendencies. Children and adults living in urban areas are at a greater risk of acquiring some kind of psychotic disorder.

If a person has been subject to social isolation, immigration related issues, social adversity, racial discrimination, unemployment, unhealthy work conditions, family dysfunction, etc., then there are increased chances of being prone to mental disorder in general, schizophrenia in particular.

Environment plays a more active role in designing and defining one's mental health. There were views that a healthy, wholesome and friendly environment is necessary to keep people happy mentally and physically.

Recent researches have shown surprising patterns in determining one's psychological well being. It is now a greater responsibility as parents to ensure a good environment which creates and nurtures healthy human beings.

Mental disorders have become a new menace to mankind. The rate of people suffering from psychotic disorders has been constantly rising.

Substance or drug abuse

It has been found that people with schizophrenia have a greater intake of nicotine than others. Other drugs like Cocaine, Amphetamine and to some extent alcohol are very common abuses amongst the people suffering from schizophrenia.

They have not been termed as probable causes of the disease, but the consumption level is very surprising. Alcohol is the most commonly used intoxicant with schizophrenics. With the abuse of such drugs, there are increased chances of experiencing problems which are very similar to schizophrenia.

The will power and logical sense of these subjects is quite weak. And as a result, there is a tendency to get attracted to intoxicants which aggravate their disorder.

There are times when the subjects feel so disoriented, restless and tensed that they try to get some respite through these drugs. Some find relief and others get worse.

Cannabis is another commonly used drug for those coping with the symptoms of schizophrenia. It is not a cause of the disease and cannot make a person suffer or develop schizophrenia. However, it definitely aggravates and worsens the problem.

Consumption of Cannabis is not enough to cause any psychotic disease, but its prolonged usage has been found as a contributory factor in making the cases worse than ever.

Early exposure to cannabis goes on to cause schizoaffective disorders in adult life. Excessive use of Cannabis, however, has been found as the cause of some very disturbed mental conditions.

- Drugs are mainly used by these subjects as coping mechanisms for the stress, loneliness, anxiety, depression or boredom that they feel.

Prenatal and unhealthy childhood factors

If the mother was suffering from some viral infection, hypoxia, stress, or malnutrition during fetal development, the child has greater chances of suffering from schizophrenia in adulthood.

People born in the Northern Hemisphere in summer or spring time have 6-8% more chances of being diagnosed with schizophrenia due to increased viral infections at the time of birth or early infancy.

What kind of virus play a specific role of causing this disease in childhood or adulthood? This is still a mystery. However, role of viral infections cannot be ignored.

- Low oxygen levels at the time of birth due to prolonged labor or premature birth may also cause this disease.

- Physical or sexual abuse in childhood has been found as a very common cause of this disease. Children who had undergone physical violence, beating and other tortures, or were sexually abused, molested, raped are subject to psychotic symptoms of schizophrenia later in life, or immediately after such a traumatic event has taken place.

Brain Abnormalities

Abnormal brain chemistry definitely plays a role. However, brain structure plays a very important role in schizophrenia. Deficit in the volume of brain tissues resulting from enlarged brain ventricles is seen as a very common cause.

The frontal lobe responsible for analysis, planning, reasoning, decision making, interpretation and other such faculties is very slow in its activity in such subjects. So a slow frontal lobe can cause schizophrenia.

It is highly unlikely that schizophrenia is the result of one particular abnormality in human brain in one particular area as the frontal lobe, hippocampus, amygdala were also seen in a dysfunctional state in a schizophrenic subject.

Some common mechanisms of Schizophrenia

Scientists have tried to establish a link between an alteration in brain function and schizophrenia. And the most common dysfunction is the mind's faulty interpretation of the firing of "dopaminergic neurons". This has been named "dopamine hypothesis" and this has a direct link with brain neurons and schizophrenia.

Psychological mechanisms

Those diagnosed positively for schizophrenia are seen with identifiable problems of cognitive biases under some testing or confusing circumstances. Memory loss and some other neurocognitive deficits are global and some deficits vary according to particular problems and experiences.

- There have been some recent reports that people suffering from schizophrenia respond emotionally to negative situations and stressful circumstances which makes them more vulnerable to mood and mental disorders.

- There are also reports that the nature and content of delusions are the probable causes of emotional disturbances and trauma which could have caused schizophrenia.

- The measures that such a subject undertakes to avoid the threats are indicative of the chronicity of the disease.

- There are people with minor delusions of threats and minor precautionary measures; they are not as delusional as the ones with severe threats and precautions.

Neurological mechanisms

Neural circuits of the brain are altered in schizophrenia which goes on to suggest that the disease is caused by neurodevelopmental disorders. In 40-50% of the total cases, slight brain alteration is seen.

However, it is still not clear whether these changes have always been there in the brain which could have caused the disease or they occurred due to the disease.

Brain chemistry is altered in most of the mental or neurological disorders and severe psychotic problems too. FMRI and PET, which are brain imaging technologies, have shown that people with schizophrenia have functional variations in certain parts of the brain like frontal lobe, hippocampus, temporal lobes, etc. Reduction in brain volume in the areas of frontal cortex and temporal lobes has also been seen. However, it has not been determined whether these factors pre-existed or are the developments caused by the disease itself.

The widely accepted "dopamine hypothesis" has claimed that excessive activation of D2 receptors caused Schizophrenia. This discovery was accidental once it was realized that Phenothiazine drug, which are used to control and regulate dopamine function, was helpful in controlling psychotic symptoms.

And drugs like Amphetamines which increased dopamine functions exacerbated psychotic symptoms. This accidental discovery has helped greatly in understanding the disease, causes, mechanisms and even the treatment.

Reduced glutamate functions looks like a cause of Schizophrenia as it restricts one's performance in tests, analysis, management, etc. Role of glutamate pathways has been accepted as a cause of Schizophrenia, but a very minor cause because people with positive symptoms do not respond to glutamate management medication.
All this study shows is that neurological mechanisms have a key role to play in

schizophrenia like any other neuropsychiatric disorder. However, to what extent, in what way, and for how long are still some questions which have not been answered.

Answers to these queries with more research and analysis can surely help psychologists arrive at a firmer conclusion about the role of brain in Schizophrenia.

5: Medical and Psychological Cure of Schizophrenia

Schizophrenia is very disturbing to know for some people generally because it is commonly believed that it cannot be treated. This misconception has gone very deep into the society that schizophrenia is an incurable disease and there are no chances of recovery.

That is why a positive diagnosis of this disease sounds like a death siren to most people. It devastates the subjects and his/her friends and family.

- Schizophrenic patient can live a full, normal and balanced life if it is diagnosed early in life. The symptoms will not grow worse if it is diagnosed early and recovery for schizophrenia is not impossible.

- If you suspect Schizophrenia for yourself or your loved one, see a doctor right away. The picture of recovery from this disease is not as grim and there is a lot of hope.

- It is like diabetes, there is no cure yet, but it can be managed successfully so you can remain healthy and fit with the help of medication and other supportive therapies.

If you are diagnosed with this unfortunate disease, it does not necessarily mean a life imprisonment with illness, hospitalizations etc. It will not bring an endless series of hospitalizations, bouts of illnesses, worst case of delusions and hallucinations.

Cases and subjects have shown improvement with medication generally. According to The Royal College of Psychiatrists, UK, this disease has good chances of recovery:

- 1 in 5 schizophrenia patients get better within 5 years of the diagnosis.

- 3 out of 5 improve drastically with only minor symptoms occurring from time to time from mild to severe forms.

- Only 1 in 5 will continue to have chronic and acute problems.

Schizophrenia takes lifetime to recover as it cannot be cured by antibiotics. It is a complex disorder of the brain and psychology and there is no sure shot prescription.

Even during medication, the symptoms may continue to occur from time to time and it is a challenging journey. However, wellness is a goal to be achieved for a schizophrenic and one has to keep working towards the goal. A lot of management is needed with the symptoms, needs and erratic behavior.

- A wholesome treatment regime of schizophrenia involves handling and cures of current symptoms, avoid future symptoms from taking place, restoring the ability and confidence to function like a normal person and live a good life. A treatment plan which involves medication along with psychological and emotional support system is the best.

Some heartening facts about Schizophrenia

- Schizophrenia is curable. Even when there is no cure in a specific way, this disease can be efficiently and successfully managed. Every person is treated differently depending on the illness, chronicity, symptoms, background, nature etc.

- One can enjoy a normal life. A schizophrenic can enjoy a balanced life with meaningful relationships and stability after being treated.

- Hospitalization is not your middle name. Just because you are diagnosed with this disorder does not mean you now have to be hospitalized frequently.

- Be hopeful, no matter how trying the circumstances are. Do not lose hope. Face the challenges with bravery and confidence.

How to have an effective recovery plan?

A positive attitude towards the treatment is very important. The sooner you see a doctor, better your chances of getting well and responding well to medication. As soon as you feel or see any of the symptoms we have already discussed, see a psychiatric doctor rather than your usual family doctor.

You need expert help in this and running around from pillar to post is not only going to make it worse but even harmful. If an untrained doctor administers a medicine without understanding the disease, there is a chance you may be harmed by it. Trust a professional who has experience and knowledge in these things.

Every individual is treated differently in psychiatry as no two individuals are alike. It is not a viral infection where a standard prescribed antibiotic works all the time. Treatment must be custom made according to your problems, disorders, and symptoms.

Be an active participant of the treatment plan and recovery. Your feedback, opinion, analysis, needs and concerns are very important. Make sure that you communicate these feelings with your doctor.

- The most effective way is the involvement of your friends, family, loved ones, your own self, and your therapist as part of the whole plan. Co-ordination and harmony amongst all the components is very vital.

- Your perception and thought about the treatment really matters.

- The world is full of all sorts of people and they may have different opinions about your disorder. Do not allow anybody to make you feel miserable or inferior because of your problems. Refuse to give in to their tactics of making you small or bad.

  It is good to take your illness seriously. However, do not allow yourself to drown in this myth of "never getting better," or "life is over". Associate with people who value you for the person that you are and look beyond your diagnosed disorder.

  Hang out with your friends and family who love you and support you.

- Feel free to communicate with your therapist. It is your doctor's duty to treat you and your doctors know best whether a particular drug is helping you or not.

Dosage should not be too much or too little. There has to be a balance or you will get knocked off your senses due to an overdose, and under dose may not show any results.

Tell your doctor how you feel about the treatment. Your opinion should be paid special attention. If you do not have faith in the therapist or the treatment you are receiving, you will not respond well to the drugs administered by the doctor. Ask questions if you have any side effects, long term-short term perspective etc.

- Mere medication and drugs are not going to help much. You need to have some supportive theories, learn to ignore or cut the chatter of the mind, stop believing in delusions and tell yourself that they are a creation of the mid without any actual existence. Start believing that you'll get well and that you are safe and loved.

- Set some meaningful goals for yourself. Get involved with society and community and make yourself useful rather than being depressed.

Effective support system can turn things around. Emotional and psychological support system is necessary, along with medication. Request your friends and family to be co-operative with you. Tell them that they are an important part of your life and you may call upon them in times of distress and need.

They'll surely be happy to help. Build trust and faith in yourself and treat them well. They are most likely to hold your hands through the journey and bring out the best in you. Engage with people who bring out the best in you and make you feel important and dignified.

- Try to stay involved with others. There are urges for a person suffering from schizophrenia to be isolated or reclusive. Kick that urge away and come out of your shell. Go out, dine, walk on the green grass, shop, watch TV, joke, laugh and try to live a normal life and forget that you are diagnosed with schizophrenia.

If you continue with your life thinking that you are ill and that you are worthless, believe me, it wrecks havoc. Kick the illness and its thoughts aside, but be honest with yourself.

- Volunteer for social work. Do what you love to do. Paint, sketch, social work, pray, play, join community service, church service, or anything else that keeps you happy.

- Look for the options available in your local area about mental health clinics, hospitals, rejuvenation centers etc. Participate in them.

Being around loved ones is very effective in recovery according to research and reports. If you have a co-operative family that understands the illness well and is ready to contribute towards your wellness, there is nothing like it. Make use of the opportunity and get rid of substance abuse, if there is any.

Healthy lifestyle choices

Some people suffer more than others in schizophrenia. Make yourself competent to manage stress. This will not only keep you well but also empower you and help you build self confidence. If you are ready to help yourself, you won't be hopeless and helpless.

- Learn to manage stress because stress can really make the situation worse in schizophrenia. Do not over work and make sure you get enough rest. Always find a way to relax if you are feeling disturbed.

- Avoid caffeine and exercise regularly. This helps you relax, burn energy and sleep well. You really need to get a lot of sleep and standard 6-7 hours may not be enough.

- Avoid drugs and alcohol. People taking any kind of intoxicants stand a greater chance of making their condition worse.

- Undertake a fitness regimen, go to gym, walk, run, jog or do yoga. It helps in keeping the body and mind fit. It has dual benefits.

- Find things to do that make you feel confident. Cultivate a sense of dignity and prestige and start practicing a hobby or passion regularly. It will fulfill you with a sense of accomplishment.

Medication has a place of its own

You cannot depend totally on medication, as medication is not a cure for your disease. It is just a remedy to manage and control the symptoms through psychotic drugs. Hallucinations, delusions, fear, anger and depression etc., is handled through these drugs and they are not capable of curing them by any standards.

It can treat some of the symptoms of schizophrenia effectively but not all of them. Social withdrawal, lack of motivation, inability to express emotions cannot be controlled or regulated by drugs. They need counseling, emotional and psychological help.

Some drugs or therapies may have disturbing side effects. They may be drowsiness, weakness, loss of energy, uncontrolled movements, sexual dysfunction, and weight gain/loss. Such side effects may be varying in their intensity and if you or your family members are being bothered and worried about all this, speak to your doctor. Probable dosage may need to be reduced or your medications need to be switched.

There may be trials with the medication that suits you best and this may take some time to arrive at a final prescription.

- If you are being bothered or disturbed with the medicines, do not stop or reduce on your own. Speak to you therapist first. Making the decision yourself without doctor's advice may be harmful to you.

How to find the right medication?

It may take some time to figure out which medicine work and which medicine don't work. There have been patterns where some symptoms of schizophrenia take a long time to disappear. In some people, it disappears in few days.

There have been cases where a patient responded positively to the medication within 4-6 weeks. They determine the kind of improvement or change they are going to bring to a person's psychological health.

Anti-psychotics show remarkable development and improvement in positive symptoms. However, they have not been found very effective in negative symptoms and cognitive dysfunction. There haven't been many evidence of consistent improvement beyond a period of two - three years.

The choice of psychotics is based on the analysis of cost, benefits, and risks. There are two categories of psychotic drugs, "typical" or the old drugs and "atypical" or the latest drugs.

- Typical drugs are not used frequently now because of the neurological disorders associated with them as side effects, which are commonly known as "extra pyramidal symptoms".

These symptoms could be any of these:

Restlessness, pacing, extremely slow movements and thoughts, altered breathing and heart rate, muscle spasms of back or legs, temporary paralysis, tremors and shocks, muscle stiffness etc.

There is another big threat caused by typical drugs and that is "tardive dyskinesia", which is the involuntary movement of tongue or mouth, hands, feet, etc.

According to the reports published by National Alliance on Mental Illness, with every passing year there is an increase of 5% in the risk of developing tardive dyskinesia with the usage of typical drugs.

- Atypical drugs are now used as the latest medicines because the side effects associated with them are not as grave at the level of neurological disturbances. They have side effects, like loss of motivation, weight gain, sexual dysfunction, depression, nervousness, drowsiness, or sedation.

Both classes have their own side effects. If used for a long time, it has not been proven to be beneficial for overall well being. Both have similar drop-out rates and relapses as it has been noticed. They both have 40-50% positive response if administered at low or moderate levels, 30-40% show only partial improvement and 20% show no change.

There is no fixed set to be followed which ensures success and improvement. "*Clozapine*" has been used very effectively on patients who have not shown any response to typical and atypical drugs. They fall in the category of "treatment resistant" or "refractory" schizophrenia.

This drug has a fatal side effect of decreasing white blood cell count in almost 4% of the cases. On one hand, where typical drugs have neurological side effects, atypical have metabolic syndrome. It is yet to be proven whether these new psychotic drugs cause "neuroleptic malignant syndrome," which is a very rare but fatal neurological disorder.

The American Psychiatric Association suggests stopping all medication if no symptoms of schizophrenia are found for one year.

Some commonly used typical antipsychotic drugs are:

Chlorpromazine, Fluphenazine, Haloperidol, Loxapine, Molindone, Perphenanzine, Thioridazine, Thiothixene.

Some atypical psychotic drugs are:

Aripiprazole, ozapine, Iloperidone, Olanzapine, Paliperidone, Quetiapine, Risperidone, Ziprasidone.

Facilities

There is help available for US citizens and in other countries who offer some kind of social security for unemployed, disabled, or sick people. This ensures basic life necessities like housing, clothing, food and medical expenses. There are two types of social security available in the US - SSI and SSD, which have two categories of people covered under it.

Other than this, there are residential care centers for those undergoing psychotic episodes. They either need critical care or are a disturbance or threat to others. There are rehab centers too for those who are cured or are doing better but still need training and guidance for a normal life.

Other facilities include sharing an apartment for those who can manage on their own and respond well to medication. They have help and support available nearby with trained professionals.

Prevention is better than cure

Research has shown that if some prenatal care and precautions are taken, there may be a chance to reduce the risk of schizophrenia. There are no definite dos and don'ts.
Viral infections during pregnancy, stress, and trauma should be avoided as this may ensure better resistance and lesser chances of suffering from schizophrenia.

Some viral infections really cause a lot of stress, disturbance and problems during pregnancy. Nutrition also plays a key role for the mother during pregnancy.

Two things have come out of the reports, *omega 3* fish oils and prenatal *Choline*. These supplements have been found very useful and reliable for developing and giving birth to intelligent and mentally balanced children. High level *Choline* (a vitamin B group nutrient) intake during pregnancy makes the child have healthy brain as they "charge baby brains".

Omega 3 fatty acids have also been found very helpful in eliminating the chances of schizophrenia along with other psychotic disorders.

- There are no set standards for treating and preventing schizophrenia. However, if some precautions are taken and certain good things are ensured, we can truly fight this disease or at least delay it, make it less chronic and disturbing.

6: Love and Support to Help Your Loved One Recover

Love, support and help for a schizophrenia patient are very important. It helps greatly in treatment and recovery. One can really do a great and huge contribution by being co-operative, loving and understanding towards the patient.

With proper medication, recovery from this dreadful disorder is not just a possibility but a reality. Dealing with a family member with schizophrenia may be difficult for anybody, but you do not have to take the whole responsibility on your own shoulders. Make others participate. Ask friends, relatives or seek help from community or church.

The first thing to do while helping your loved one struggling with the disorder is to learn to accept the disease. You may be dealing with a lot of abnormal behavior, and there may be a feeling of fear, guilt, frustration, anger, embarrassment, helplessness and hopelessness in your heart.

You may feel very helpless to see your loved one's miserable condition. To see them suffering is a very painful sight. There are some social factors that may disturb you, like the stigma of schizophrenia or any mental disorder, the fear of losing your reputation, dignity and respect.

There may be times when you want to hide the patient and yourself to escape an unpleasant situation or ridicule.

- First accept the disease and the problems that come along with it. Try to be a sport and take the problems lightly, try to laugh off the stress.

- Be realistic about the expectations that you have from such a patient. Do not expect miraculous changes. Make the patient feel good and confident about him/her.

- Do not lose hope and look forward to a better situation. Enjoy life with normalcy.

Tips for family members

A helping family member has to educate himself/herself about the disease. Speak to a therapist, read books, journals, etc., to prepare you in order to travel on the road to recovery. It'll enable you to handle the illness, its troubles, and the setbacks.

- Reduce stress in the atmosphere and do not force the patient to recover. It is not under his/her control. A stressful situation not only makes the patient uncomfortable but also the other members from trying to live a normal life.

- Be realistic about the speed and outcomes of the treatment process. Do not expect the person to improve overnight. It builds disappointment, irritation and hopelessness.

- Do not overdo the help and support mechanism. This makes the person more ill and unsure about himself/herself.

Encourage them and motivate them. Do not run all over the house as if the world is on fire, trying to help them even with the smallest of things. Give them easy responsibilities which are easy to accomplish and makes them feel important and happy.

This depends a lot on the stage and chronicity of the disease. Some people are more capable than others.

Look after yourself

If you want the support system to be effective and long lasting, take some time for yourself. Look after your health and fitness. Find some healthy ways to keep you fit and cope with the difficult situations.

- You cannot take care of anything properly if you are feeling helpless, unloved, and unimportant. You need love, encouragement and care in order to look after the patient. Have your own support system; mingle with people who understand you.

- Join a family support group. There are people who have already experienced and handled what you are going through. Take the time to talk and exchange ideas. It will help both ways.

Nobody understands better than somebody who has lived it or seen it. This helps build some emergency support system too. You can call upon them in time of need. They will surely help you.

There have been times when such patients have responded psychologically and emotionally to people they meet at such meetings. And also make friends. It is very beneficial.

- Spare some time for yourself and do what you love to do. Pursue a hobby or a passion. Exercise, walk, read, paint, go out, shop, watch a movie, cook, or just pick up anything which works like a stress buster for you.

- Take good care of your health, sleep well and eat healthy. Do not lose your appetite and sleep over this disorder. You need to stay on top of any medical condition.

- It is not necessary that you make friends only with people associated with the disease. Have people in your life who take you away from all that. Stealing some time to have a normal life is not a sin. You surely do not want to end up in an asylum yourself. You have a life of your own and never shy away from indulging.

Why is it so important to manage stress?

Schizophrenia is a disorder that makes people supporting the patient very stressed and helpless. It is a problem that keeps testing your patience night in and night out..

If you are not in a position to manage your own stress levels, you are bound to get irate, edgy, and overwhelmed. If you are not in a balanced state, you will build up a stressful environment and end up disturbing the patient too.

- Give up the attitude as if you are the only sufferer in the universe and your life has been ruined by God. You are not the only person who has been chosen to suffer. The "why me?" mindset makes things worse.

Life is not being unfair to you. Do not keep fussing about the troubles. Accept things the way they are. Do not go on defining your life with all your negativity and troubles.

- The happiest people are not those who have the least troubles. The happiest people are those people who learn to find joy in difficult circumstances. You have to find joy, take time to share a joke, laugh and be happy.

- Know what you are capable of doing and what you are not. No point getting worked up or exhausted if you take too much on your head. If you cannot handle the stress, look for alternatives.

- Do not take any blame for the illness or disorder if you have not been a direct cause. If the patient is not recovering fast or responding to medicines, it is not your fault. Do not feel guilty. These things are not within your control.

What you can control or manage is already being done by you, to care for your loved one. It is very important to encourage and motivate your loved one. The hardest thing that friends and family have to face is to convince their loved one to see a doctor for their illness.

They do not accept that there is something wrong with them because the world they are living in is perfect. They cannot find anything wrong with it. They are also afraid of the stigma, ridicule and disrespect that come with it.

The most important thing you can do is to make your loved one stick to medication. They have a tendency to skip it or discontinue. People who are undergoing delusions and hallucinations are the most difficult to convince. They have their own theories that they are being poisoned; there are threats to their life, or something else.

If they feel threatened by a family member, then it is almost impossible to convince them of their disease or your noble intentions. You may have to find some alternative ways to administer medicines. However, it is best to treat them and inform them about it.

- If the patient is apprehensive or unsure about a family member, give him/her some respite. Keep that person away from direct interaction. Do not take them to the doctor along with the patient. Give them an option to choose a doctor of their choice if they feel that they are in a commanding position.

- Some people are hesitant to see a doctor because they are afraid of being labeled as "mad" or "crazy". Tell them that you will not discuss the schizophrenia symptoms but will talk about more general problems, such as insomnia, loss of appetite, etc. This may build some confidence.

Monitor medication

Once your loved one has agreed to see a doctor, you have accomplished some success. Now, do not leave him/her to medication and think that your job is over. Your responsibility is still the same as it used to be.

Keep a close watch on the side effects. They need to be taken very seriously. Whatever disturbing side effects occur, bring it to the doctor's attention. The doctor may be able to reduce the dosage, switch medication or even reduce the harmful effects to some extent.

- You have to motivate your loved one to take medication regularly and believe that it will help them.

- Be careful that the person does not indulge in drugs and alcohol as we have already discussed.

- Keep a regular track of your loved one's progress and reports. See the doctor once in a while to discuss the issues and keep him informed of all the details.

Watch for indications showing a relapse

Most of the relapses take place due to discontinued medication. There is a good chance that as soon as the medication is discontinued without doctor's advice, relapse may occur, or the case may turn for the worse.

Many people feel that if their schizophrenia is stable or is not causing any major trouble, they should discontinue the medication. This is not recommended without the doctor's consent. However, it is advisable to be under some kind of medication if they want to keep those symptoms at bay.

Ask your doctor about the signs of relapse and look for them. There may be times when psychotic symptoms increase or worsen even during medication. You have to be watchful about those symptoms. They are quite similar to the psychotic disorders which led to the diagnosis of the disease and if you recognize the early signs of relapse, you may be able to avert a major emergency situation.

- If you notice any relapses or signs like social withdrawal, insomnia, nonsense talks, hallucinations, delusions, or paranoia, call the doctor right away. The person needs medical attention immediately.

Always be prepared for a crisis

Even after you have taken all the necessary steps, if the condition of the patient weakens or deteriorates drastically, get help from family, friends and others as you may need to hospitalize the person right away.

Keep a list of doctors, emergency care and critical care for such situations. Be prepared to have some family or friends available immediately to look after your dependants while you are fighting with the crisis.

How to handle a person with schizophrenia

- Do not try to talk reason or logic with a psychotic person

- Do not be sarcastic or shout at them in anger

- The person probably is already scared and terrified with his/her loss of sanity

- Decrease the volume of the TV, music or any other distractions

- Avoid continuous eye contact and do not stare

- Do not touch them all the time; they may not like being touched

Give the person a comfortable place to live

After being diagnosed with the disease, it is very important to decide if the family wants to live with the person. Dealing with schizophrenia could be difficult if there are children or elderly people at home.

If living under the same roof brings problems to the family, you might consider putting the patient in health care centers or hospitals.
Living with family is a very good option to exercise, but not at the cost of other's health and

well-being. It could be done only if there are no vulnerable members in the family or the support system is good.

- If a person is violent, aggressive, addicted to alcohol or drugs, then staying at home is not a very sensible options as the person needs more than love and care. They need an expert supervision.

If a person stays at home, he has a friendly environment and may agree to join activities which will help in recovery. With the help of others, a relaxed environment could be created at home.

- Being at home may not be advisable if there are elders and children who are being bothered. It will cast a negative influence on the kids. It is also not advisable if the whole family is just going crazy about the patient, or the support system of the family is not as dependable. If any of these factors are there, find an alternative.

- Do not feel guilty if you are unable to accommodate the person in your house. You have to look after other members of your family as you have equal responsibility towards them.

Contact the local mental hospitals or take advice from your doctor about the residential treatment facilities in your areas. There are institutions that provide very good care and cure to such patients. Find one close to your residence so that you may be able to visit anytime.

- 24 hour treatment facility is good for those whose psychotic symptoms are acute and need a lot of supervision and care.

- There are other options like a transitional group home which basically involves skills training and personality development, along with medication.

- Boarding houses are also an option where people who can look after themselves, people who have considerable independence. Here, they can lead a near normal life. They provide basic needs like food, shelter, etc., and the life there is quite independent.

- Some institutions provide apartments within the medical facility center to people who are functioning well with medication. Since there are only minor disturbances, they can either get an apartment for themselves or share it with other people. And of course help is available immediately in times of need. Being in a state of fear about the loved one is very common as there are threats to his/her life, sanity and normalcy. However, this road is not as gloomy as it looks.

Do not get devastated with the news. It is just another disorder and a positive outlook is necessary. There is no point in worrying and fretting about the patient when you should conserve your energy to take care of them. Life for you or him/her is not over.

7: Prognosis of Schizophrenia

Schizophrenia causes people to suffer from various other disorders like obesity, sedentary life, smoking, drugs and alcohol abuse.

It is a major factor for causing some kind of physical, mental and psychological disability. Almost three-fourths of the people suffering from Schizophrenia continue to have a disability of some kind, which definitely makes the picture grim.

However, people do come to live and function comfortably after they have the condition well managed through medication. People in developing countries have fared much better in recovering and improving than the ones in undeveloped ones.

This has been heartening news for people in the Third World countries as their medical facilities are not as competent or advanced, and there is mass illiteracy and poverty.

Life expectancy in Schizophrenic people is quite low due to high suicide rates along with other diseases. This makes it a disorder with a high human cost.

Medication helps but prolonged medication has also been seen to cause or aggravate the psychotic symptoms or the hallucinations and delusions. The side effects of medication are numerous even with the latest drugs, and the series of hospitalization increases the economic cost.

There have been people who have fought against heavy odds to conquer or at least manage this disorder and lived a very successful and goal-oriented life.

- We all have heard of Dr. John Forbes Nash Jr. who was honored with the Noble Prize for economics, one of the greatest mathematicians of the modern times, suffered from Schizophrenia.

He has the mind of a genius along with Schizophrenic delusions and hallucinations. He has been successful in managing his disorder very efficiently and continued with his ground breaking research.

He struggled with delusions that the government agents were out to persecute him. His life became the inspiration for the Academy Awards Winner movie, A Beautiful Mind, which depicts his story.

- Who doesn't know Peter Green, the famous guitarist and his signature sound, who was also a founding member of the Fleetwood Mac. He struggled with violent episodes of Schizophrenia, spent years in psychiatric hospitals and was recluse for many years. He later started recovering and has managed his disorder well and performs at live shows now.

- Lionel Aldridge helped the Green Bay Packers win two super bowls and stayed in the NFL for ten glorious years. He retired from football and few years later developed Schizophrenia, continued to struggle with it for a long time and finally succeeded in gaining a balanced state.

After this, he gave his life to help and advocate for the homeless and the mentally disturbed.

- Brian Wilson, a former leader of the Beach Boys and a Grammy award winner singer, became one of the greatest singers of all times in the Rolling Stones' ranking. He developed schizoaffective disorder and started hearing sounds and had delusions.

Many theories came out as probable causes of his disorder, drug abuse and heart condition being the most common. He suffered from many psychotic disorders but never gave up his fight. He is now in a balanced state, performs on stage and has a fan following.

- Syd Barret and Mary Todd Lincoln were also suspected of suffering from Schizophrenia but the cases were not reported formally.

- Some other notable names who suffered some form of Schizophrenia, out of which, few lucky ones refused to give up and conquered, while others succumbed or could not make it.

Buddy Bolden (jazz musician), Clara Bow (Hollywood actress), Parveen Babi (Indian actress), Eduard Einstein (son of Albert Einstein), Vincent van Gogh (visual artist, painter), Jim Gordon (drummer), Tom Harrell (jazz musician), Adele Hugo (daughter of French writer victor Hugo, her life has been portrayed in a film named the story of Adele), Rufus May (clinical psychologist), Katherine Routledge (British archaeologist), John Ogdon (English pianist and composer), Jeremy Oxley (musician and member of Australian band

the Sunnyboys), William Chester Minor
(contributed to the Oxford English Dictionary).

These are the names which were famous. There are
many who came out victorious and overcame this
disease while others were not as famous and died
unsung.

Conclusion

I hope that this book has succeeded in its goal of spreading awareness about this "misunderstood and dreaded" disorder. Schizophrenia is a disorder associated with the psychology and brain and it is not life threatening or impossible to manage, contrary to the general conception about this disease. If some precautions are taken, and some other factors are well managed and understood, this disorder can be prevented to a great extent.

Life does not end with Schizophrenia and this is the message that this book wants to convey. This book was written not to scare you or tell you heartening lies about this condition but to inform you and educate you on what this disorder is about.

Have faith and confidence if you have a loved one suffering from Schizophrenia, do not give up. Be aware, hopeful and confident. Differentiate between necessary Dos and fear based actions. Look after yourself and your loved ones.

CPSIA information can be obtained
at www.ICGtesting.com
Printed in the USA
LVHW021915170423
744577LV00021B/505